Sleep Oasis

Sleep Oasis:

Meditation and Mindfulness Practices for Restful Sleep and Deep Relaxation

Bruce P. Frye

Dedication

To my loved ones,

Thank you for your support on my journey to find restful sleep and deep relaxation. This book is dedicated to you. Your understanding, encouragement, and presence have meant the world to me.

And to you, my readers, I am truly grateful. Your curiosity and willingness to explore new paths have inspired me to delve deeper into the world of meditation and mindfulness. My hope is that the techniques and practices shared in this book will guide you toward inner peace and a sanctuary of tranquility.

Together, let's embark on this transformative journey, finding balance between the demands of the modern world and the rejuvenation of our bodies and minds.

Chapter 1

Introduction

Do you struggle to acquire a decent night's sleep? Is it tough for you to unwind and rest after a busy day? If so, you're not alone. In today's fast-paced and demanding environment, finding solitude and achieving deep

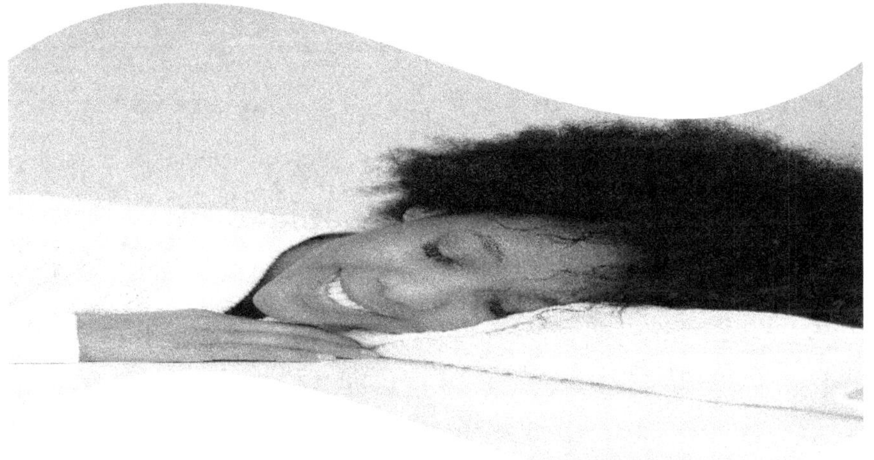

sleep can be a continuous challenge. That's why I am delighted to introduce to you the updated edition of my eBook, "Meditation and Mindfulness Practices for Better Sleep and Relaxation."

Sleep and relaxation are crucial for our general physical and mental well-being. They provide us with the opportunity to refresh and revitalize our bodies and brains, equipping us to confront the everyday obstacles and embrace the opportunities that each new day presents. Regrettably, the demands of modern life frequently make it impossible to acquire the restorative slumber we desperately need.

The effects of insufficient sleep and relaxation are far-reaching, including a spectrum of health concerns such as obesity, diabetes, cardiovascular disease, and depression. Additionally, our cognitive capabilities can be affected, impairing memory, attention, and decision-making ability. In essence, skipping appropriate sleep and relaxation might have significant effects for our holistic well-being.

Conversely, prioritizing and getting sufficient quality sleep and relaxation bestows an assortment of benefits. These include boosting our mood, enhancing our productivity, and minimizing the risk of chronic health conditions. It is apparent that making sleep and relaxation a vital issue in our lives is indispensable for keeping physical and mental health, as well as reaching our ambitions.

In this updated edition of "Meditation and Mindfulness Practices for Better Sleep and Relaxation," we will examine transformative strategies and practices that address the problems of getting deep rest and relaxation. By combining meditation and mindfulness into your everyday routine, you will uncover strong techniques to unwind, soothe your mind, and welcome deep sleep.

Get ready to embark on a revitalizing voyage of self-discovery as we delve into practical exercises, step-by-step directions, and insightful coaching. Together, we will develop a sanctuary of quiet and learn to negotiate the difficulties of the modern world while nourishing our sleep and relaxation.

Join me in understanding the keys to restful sleep and profound relaxation. Let us go on this transforming path toward improved sleep and inner tranquility.

1.1 The Power of Restful Sleep and Deep Relaxation

Restful sleep and deep relaxation are tremendously potent for our overall well-being and quality of life. They play a key role in sustaining physical, mental, and emotional wellness. Let's discuss the benefits and necessity of healthy sleep and deep relaxation.

1. Physical Restoration: During sleep, our bodies undergo critical processes of repair, renewal, and growth. Restful sleep supports muscle and tissue repair, enhances the immune system, and helps control hormones important for appetite, metabolism, and growth. It is also associated to a lower risk of chronic problems such as obesity, diabetes, cardiovascular diseases, and immunological disorders.

2. Mental Clarity and Cognitive Functioning: Quality sleep boosts cognitive capacities, memory consolidation, and learning. Deep sleep stages, notably REM (Rapid Eye Movement) sleep, are connected with memory consolidation and problem-solving skills. Getting sufficient restful sleep enhances focus, attention span, decision-making, creativity, and general mental performance.

3. Emotional Well-being: Sleep and relaxation have a tremendous impact on emotional control and mental health. Adequate sleep helps stabilize mood, lowers irritation, and enhances emotional resilience. On the other side, sleep deprivation is associated to increased sensitivity to stress, anxiety, depression, and mood disorders.

4. Stress Reduction: Deep relaxation, whether through meditation, mindfulness, or other practices, stimulates the body's relaxation response and counteracts the effects of chronic stress. Regular practice of relaxation techniques can lower blood pressure, reduce muscle tension, moderate heart rate, and decrease stress hormone levels. It produces a sense of relaxation and inner peace, supporting emotional balance and better general well-being.

5. Enhanced Productivity and Performance: Rested persons are more alert, focused, and invigorated, leading to higher productivity and better performance in various areas of life. Whether it's at work, school, or daily duties, having sufficient restful sleep and engaging in relaxation practices helps boost performance and efficiency.

6. Immune System Support: Sleep plays a critical role in immune function, with evidence suggesting that insufficient sleep might damage the immune system's ability to fight off infections and diseases. Prioritizing restful sleep can contribute to a stronger immune system, reducing the risk of infections and boosting general health.

Tips for Promoting Restful Sleep and Deep Relaxation:

1. Establish a regular sleep schedule: Go to bed and wake up at consistent times, including on weekends, to regulate your body's internal clock.

2. Create a sleep-friendly environment: Make your bedroom pleasant, quiet, dark, and cool. Consider utilizing earplugs, eye masks, or white noise machines to minimize interruptions.

3. Adopt a bedtime routine: Engage in soothing activities before bed, such as reading, having a warm bath, practicing relaxation techniques, or listening to quiet music.

4. Limit exposure to electronic devices: The blue light emitted by displays might interfere with sleep. Avoid using electronic gadgets for at least an hour before bed or use blue light filters.

5. Avoid stimulants: Limit caffeine and nicotine intake, especially close to bedtime, as these can alter sleep patterns.

6. Regular physical activity: Engaging in moderate exercise during the day can improve sleep quality. However, avoid strenuous exercise close to bedtime since it may excite you and make it harder to fall asleep.

7. Practice relaxation techniques: Explore various relaxation techniques such as deep breathing exercises, meditation, progressive muscle relaxation, or guided imagery to induce calm and prepare your mind and body for sleep.

Remember, prioritizing adequate sleep and deep relaxation is vital for your overall health and well-being. If you routinely battle with sleep disorders or have concerns about your sleep quality, it is essential to visit a healthcare expert for further evaluation and guidance.

1.2 Exploring Meditation and Mindfulness for Optimal Sleep and Relaxation

Meditation and mindfulness are strong activities that can greatly boost sleep quality and promote profound relaxation. They help relax the mind, alleviate stress and anxiety, and promote a sense of peace. Here's how you might explore meditation and mindfulness for better sleep and relaxation:

1. Mindful Breathing: Focus your attention on your breath. Sit or lie down comfortably and take calm, deep breaths. Notice the sensation of the breath entering and leaving your body. If your mind wanders, softly bring your attention back to the breath. This technique can help relax your body and quiet your thoughts, preparing you for comfortable sleep.

2. Body Scan Meditation: Lie down in a comfortable posture and bring your awareness to different regions of your body, starting from your toes and gently working upward. Notice any sensations, tightness, or discomfort. As you bring focus to each body part, intentionally relax and release any tension you may be carrying. This practice helps remove bodily tension and promotes profound relaxation.

3. Guided Imagery: Listen to guided imagery or visualization exercises designed to take you to a tranquil and calming place. Close your eyes, listen to the instructions, and envision yourself in a calm place such as a beach, forest, or garden. Engaging your senses in the imagery can produce a deep sense of relaxation and peace.

4. Loving-Kindness Meditation: This technique involves producing sentiments of love, kindness, and compassion towards oneself and others. Sit comfortably, close your eyes, and silently repeat mantras such as "May I be happy, may I be healthy, may I be peaceful." Then extend these wishes to loved ones, acquaintances, and even challenging persons. This practice cultivates a good and tranquil frame of mind, enabling improved sleep and relaxation.

5. Mindfulness-Based Stress Reduction (MBSR): MBSR is a systematic program that includes mindfulness meditation, bodily awareness, and gentle exercise. It focuses on increasing moment-to-moment mindfulness and non-judgmental acceptance of ideas, emotions, and bodily sensations. Participating in an MBSR program or employing MBSR practices can help reduce stress and enhance sleep quality.

6. Establishing a Bedtime Ritual: Incorporate mindfulness or meditation into your bedtime routine. Create a ritual where you set aside a few minutes before night for a soothing activity. This signals to your mind and body that it's time to unwind and prepare for sleep. You can combine moderate stretching, deep breathing, or a short meditation session to aid shift into a relaxed state.

7. Mindful Sleep: Bring mindfulness into your sleep itself. As you lie in bed, practice being totally present and sensitive to the sensations of lying down, the weight of your body on the mattress, and the feeling of the sheets against your skin. Let go of all ideas or worries, and simply focus on the current moment. This practice can help quiet a restless mind and produce a more tranquil sleep experience.

Remember, meditation and mindfulness are abilities that develop with practice. Consistency is crucial, so aim for regular workouts, even if they are brief. Experiment with several ways and see what resonates with you the most. Over time, you'll likely experience enhanced relaxation, improved sleep quality, and a stronger sense of well-being.

Chapter 2

The Art of Body Scan Meditation

The Art of Body Scan Meditation is a practice that helps you to create profound relaxation and heightened awareness by deliberately bringing your attention to different parts of your body. By gently scanning and accepting the sensations, tensions, and emotions present in each location, you build a profound connection between your mind and body. This simple yet powerful meditation technique promotes relaxation, self-awareness, and an overall sense of well-being. Through the Art of Body Scan Meditation, you can embark on a journey of self-discovery and find consolation in the present moment.

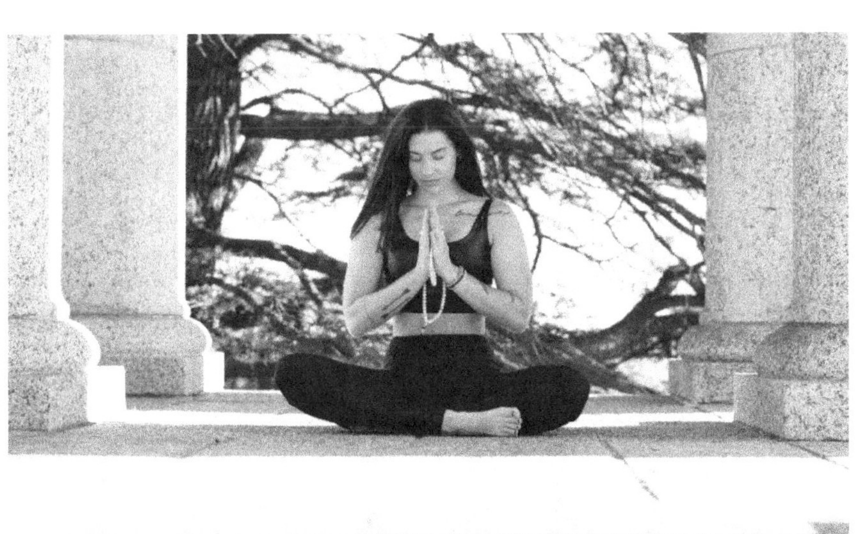

2.1 Tranquility: Body Scan Meditation for Deep Relaxation

Welcome to the practice of body scan meditation, a journey to deep relaxation and calm. In this meditation, we will gradually direct our attention through each region of the body, building a profound sense of peace and awareness. Find a comfortable posture, either sitting or lying down, and let's begin.

Take a moment to settle into your body, letting any tension or restlessness dissipate. Close your eyes if you feel comfortable doing so, and direct your attention to your breath. Take a big breath in, and as you exhale, let go of any remaining worries or distractions.

Now, move your concentration to your feet. Notice the sensation of your feet touching the earth or the support beneath you. Direct your focus to the toes, the arches, and the heels. Observe any sensations present in your feet—warmth, coolness, tingling, or any other feelings. Simply watch without judgment.

Moving up to your lower legs, bring your awareness to the calves and shins. Scan through each area, detecting any spots of tension or relaxation. Allow your breath to flow naturally as you continue to explore these sensations, noting and accepting whatever happens.

Now, focus your attention on your knees and thighs. Feel the weight and support of your legs against the surface you're lying on. Notice any sensations of warmth or coldness in this area. If you feel any discomfort or tightness, gently breathe into it, letting it soften and dissolve.

Bring your awareness to your hips and pelvis. Observe any sensations of tension or relaxation in this location. Notice the link between your breath and the small motions in your body as you continue to relax and let go.

Continue scanning your focus through your lower abdomen, your lower back, and up into your upper back and chest. Notice the rise and fall of your breath in this place and any emotions of expansion or release. Allow your breath to bring you deeper into a state of calm.

Now, bring your concentration to your hands and arms. Observe the sensations in your palms, fingers, wrists, and forearms. Notice any tension melting away as you softly breathe into these places, providing a sensation of relaxation and ease.

Move your attention to your shoulders, neck, and throat. Let go of any stress or tightness you may be holding in these regions, allowing them to soften and relax. Feel the subtle release with each breath.

Finally, bring your focus to your head and face. Notice any feelings in your scalp, forehead, eyes, cheeks, jaw, and lips. Allow these areas to relax completely, releasing any leftover tension or thoughts.

Take a moment to absorb the sense of peace that fills your entire body. Feel the deep relaxation and the connection between your mind and body. Breathe in this feeling of calmness, allowing it to nourish you from inside.

When you are ready, gently bring your focus back to the present moment. Wiggle your fingers and toes, and slowly open your eyes. Take this sensation of tranquility with you as you resume your day, knowing that you may return to this practice whenever you desire deep relaxation and quiet.

May you carry this sense of peace with you throughout your journey. Remember that the practice of body scan meditation is always open to you, creating a sanctuary of deep relaxation and self-awareness.

As you continue to explore the practice of body scan meditation, you may notice subtle modifications in your body and mind. With each session, you acquire a deeper ability to listen to your body's needs, nurturing them with care and understanding.

In this practice, the body becomes a gateway to the present moment, letting you escape the grasp of worries, anxieties, and thoughts about the past or future. Instead, you anchor your focus on the sensations that come in each instant, appreciating the wisdom and intelligence of your body.

Through body scan meditation, you learn to befriend your body, creating a greater connection with and appreciation for its intricacies. As you walk through different sections of your body, you may find areas of tension, discomfort, or emotional baggage. Rather than opposing or avoiding these sensations, allow them in with an attitude of curiosity and non-judgment.

As you advance in this technique, you may learn that the body's messages are inextricably connected with the ebb and flow of your emotions and ideas. By quietly observing and appreciating these experiences, you can build a sense of spaciousness that allows for healing and transformation.

In times of stress or restlessness, returning to the practice of body scan meditation can be a tremendous tool for self-care and renewal. By allocating frequent periods to this practice, you create a sacred space for yourself to let go, rejuvenate, and restore your energy.

Remember that this exercise is not about obtaining a specific objective or goal. It is about accepting the journey, building a loving relationship with your body, and cultivating a deep sense of calm and tranquility.

As you end this session of body scan meditation, take a few moments to express gratitude for the opportunity to connect with your body and access its inner wisdom. Carry the calm and serenity that you have cultivated into the world, sharing it with others through your presence and activities.

2.2 Unveiling the Healing Benefits of Body Scan Meditation

Body scan meditation is a practice that not only promotes deep relaxation and tranquility but also offers tremendous healing benefits for both the body and mind. Let's explore some of the ways in which this meditation approach can enhance your overall well-being and foster healing:

1. Release of Physical Tension: Through the deliberate scanning of the body, body scan meditation allows you to discover areas of physical tension or discomfort. By bringing your consciousness to these regions and actively relaxing them, you facilitate the release of built-up tension, tightness, and knots. This can help decrease physical discomfort and generate a sensation of peace and relaxation throughout your body.

2. Heightened bodily awareness: Body scan meditation cultivates a heightened feeling of bodily awareness. As you deliberately shift your attention through different portions of the body, you become attuned to subtle sensations, changes, and signals from inside. This improved awareness enables you to recognize and correct any imbalances or areas that may require care, creating a proactive attitude toward your overall physical health.

3. Emotional Healing: The body and mind are intimately connected, and emotional experiences can appear as physical sensations or tension in the body. By practicing body scan meditation, you create a safe environment to examine and process emotions that may be kept within the body. As you bring gentle awareness to these regions, you allow emotions to surface and be recognized, facilitating emotional healing and a higher sense of emotional well-being.

4. Stress Reduction: Body Scan Meditation is a wonderful tool for stress reduction. The practice asks you to slow down, relax, and let go of the accumulated stress and tension in your body and mind. By focusing your attention on each region of the body and actively releasing tension, you stimulate the body's relaxation response, which counteracts the consequences of chronic stress. Regular practice of body scan meditation can considerably lower stress levels, leading to increased general health and well-being.

5. Mind-Body Connection: Body Scan Meditation develops the mind-body connection, developing a deeper knowledge of the interplay between your ideas, emotions, and physical sensations. By examining how your mental and emotional moods develop in the body, you might get insight into the underlying causes of discomfort or imbalances. This knowledge helps you make deliberate decisions and take appropriate actions to support your overall health and wellness.

6. Improved Sleep Quality: The deep relaxation caused by body scan meditation has a direct impact on sleep quality. By carefully relaxing the body and calming the mind before sleep, you establish perfect conditions for a good night's sleep. As the body and mind unwind, sleep becomes more revitalizing, allowing for physical repair, mental restoration, and emotional recharge.

7. Mindful Living: Body Scan Meditation encourages you to be present in the moment and create awareness in your daily life. As you practice bringing focused attention to your body, you develop the capacity to be fully present and involved in each moment, free from distractions and fears. This mindfulness flows over into your interactions, activities, and decision-making, boosting your entire quality of life.

8. Increased Self-Compassion: Body Scan Meditation creates a soft and caring attitude towards yourself and your body. As you bring awareness to each part of your body, you create a sense of kindness and acceptance,

regardless of any discomfort or faults you may face. This practice develops a loving relationship with your body, fostering self-compassion, self-care, and a greater connection to your inner self.

9. Enhanced Mindfulness and Stress Management Abilities: Body Scan Meditation acts as a gateway to improving mindfulness and stress management abilities. By exercising sustained attention and non-judgmental awareness of physiological sensations, you enhance your ability to be present and grounded in the midst of daily problems. This skill set allows you to negotiate challenging situations with better resilience and clarity, boosting your overall mental well-being.

10. Holistic Wellness Integration: Body Scan Meditation blends many dimensions of wellness—physical, mental, emotional, and spiritual—into a single experience. It emphasizes a holistic approach to health and well-being, realizing that true healing entails nurturing all areas of your being. By engaging in this practice, you go on a path of self-discovery, personal growth, and wholeness.

11. Mind-Body Stress Release: Stress and tension often accumulate in the body, leading to a range of physical and mental health difficulties. Body scan meditation is a strong tool for stress release by bringing conscious awareness to the regions where tension manifests. As you observe and release tension via the exercise, you encourage the discharge

of stress from the body, resulting in a sense of lightness, relaxation, and overall well-being.

12. Improved Focus and Concentration: Regular practice of body scan meditation strengthens your capacity to focus and concentrate. By training your attention to travel systematically through different bodily areas, you acquire mental discipline and enhance your capacity to sustain attention in the present moment. This focused attention can be extended to other areas of your life, enhancing productivity, clarity, and overall cognitive performance

13. Emotional Resilience: Body Scan Meditation cultivates emotional resilience by allowing you to meet and accept emotions with compassionate awareness. As you examine the emotions that come up during the practice, you build the skill to be present and open to the full spectrum of emotions without becoming overwhelmed or reacting. This resilience fosters emotional well-being and helps you navigate life's adversities with greater serenity.

14. Overall Well-being and Life Balance: The restorative advantages of body scan meditation extend beyond specific components of health. As you apply this practice to your life, you develop a harmonious balance between your physical, mental, and emotional well-being. This integration enhances overall vitality, a deep sense of inner calm, and a more balanced approach to life.

Incorporating body scan meditation into your daily practice can have dramatic impacts on your overall health and well-being. As you explore the depths of this practice, you unearth the immense potential for healing and self-discovery that sits within you. Embrace the journey, be gentle with yourself, and savor the tremendous healing effects that body scan meditation brings. May your path be blessed with tranquility, rejuvenation, and healthy well-being.

2.3: A Step-by-Step Guide to Mastering Body Scan Meditation

1. Find a Comfortable Position: Start by choosing a comfortable position for your body. You can choose to sit on a cushion or chair with your back straight, or you can lie down on a comfortable surface. Make sure your body is well supported and relaxed.

2. Settle into the Present Moment: Take a few moments to settle into the present moment. Close your eyes if it feels comfortable, or ease your gaze downward. Begin with taking a few deep breaths, allowing oneself to arrive fully in the present moment, and letting go of any distractions or preoccupations.

3. Bring Awareness to the Breath: Shift your attention to your breath. Notice the natural rhythm of your breath—the inhalation and exhalation. Allow your breath to be your anchor, grounding you in the present

moment. Feel the gradual rise and fall of your abdomen or the sensation of the breath moving in and out of your nose.

4. Scan from Head to Toe: Start by focusing your attention on the top of your head. Slowly and softly scan down through your body, section by section, from head to toe. You can follow a systematic order or simply let your instincts lead you. As you direct your focus to each portion, notice any sensations, tension, or relaxation that you encounter.

5. Observe sensations with wonder: As you scan each region of your body, observe the sensations that come with a sense of wonder and non-judgment. Notice any areas of tightness, warmth, coldness, tingling, or any other sensations that capture your attention. Allow yourself to fully experience each sensation without trying to change or analyze it.

6. Soften and Release Tension: When you find regions of tension or discomfort, gently direct your breath and attention to that specific location. Imagine your breath going into that portion of your body, providing a sense of relaxation and release. With each breath, visualize the tension melting away, allowing space for relaxation and ease.

7. Stay Present and Non-Judgmental: Throughout the practice, maintain a sense of presence and non-judgment. If your mind wanders or gets caught up in thoughts, gently guide your attention back to the part of the body you are examining. Be patient and kind with yourself, recognizing that it is natural for the mind to wander.

8. Cultivate Mindful Awareness: As you proceed through the body scan, cultivate mindful awareness by monitoring the subtle changes in sensations, the interplay between different body parts, and the link between your body and breath. Stay fully present in each aspect, inviting a deep sense of connection and awareness.

9. Conclude with thanks: Once you have completed the body scan, take a few moments to express thanks for this time committed to self-care and self-discovery. Acknowledge the wisdom and resilience of your body. Gradually return your focus back to the room, softly moving your fingers and toes.

10. Integrate into Daily Life: As you continue to practice body scan meditation, seek to integrate this mindfulness into your daily life. Notice moments during the day when you can bring mindful awareness to your body and the feelings it feels. Whether it's during a stroll, while eating, or during periods of rest, create a stronger connection to your body and the current moment.

Remember, mastering body scan meditation is a journey, and each practice is an opportunity for growth and inquiry. Start with shorter sessions and progressively increase the duration as you feel more comfortable. With persistent practice and perseverance, you will develop the profound skills of self-awareness, calm, and inner healing.

Chapter 3

Harnessing Serenity with Mindful Breathing

Mindful breathing is a powerful exercise that can help you create tranquility and presence in your daily life. By turning your attention to the breath, you anchor yourself in the present moment, soothing the mind and developing a sense of inner peace. Here is a step-by-step strategy to harnessing peace with mindful breathing:

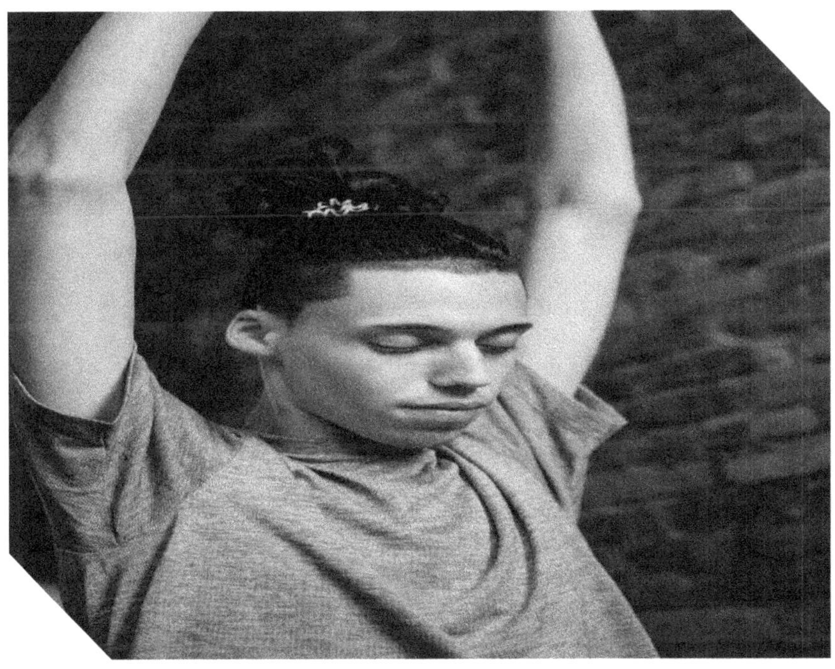

1. Find a peaceful area. Begin by finding a peaceful and comfortable area where you can sit without distractions. It might be a meditation area in your home or any spot where you can sit undisturbed for a few minutes.

2. Adopt a Comfortable Posture: Find a posture that permits you to be both relaxed and alert. You can sit cross-legged on a cushion, on a chair with your feet planted firmly on the ground, or even lie down if that is more comfortable for you. Straighten your back without straining, allowing your body to be in a natural and comfortable position.

3. Relax Your Body: Take a moment to actively relax your body. Release any tension you may be holding in your muscles, going from the top of your head down to your toes. Soften your face muscles, relax your shoulders, and let your body sink into a state of ease and relaxation.

4. Bring Attention to the Breath: Begin to transfer your focus to your breath. Notice the natural flow of your breath as it enters and departs your body. Be conscious of the sensation of the breath as it goes in and out of your nostrils, or the rise and fall of your abdomen.

5. Anchor Your Attention: Choose a precise point of attention for your breath, such as the sensation at the tip of your nose or the gentle rise and fall of your abdomen. Rest your attention on this chosen point, utilizing it as an anchor to keep your mind present.

6. Notice without judgment: As you continue to breathe, simply notice the breath without judgment or trying to modify it. Notice the nature of each breath—whether it is deep or shallow, long or brief. Allow your breath to be as it is, accepting it without resistance or expectation.

7. Gently Return to the Breath: It is common for the mind to stray during meditation. When you find that your mind has strayed away, gently and non-judgmentally return your focus back to the breath. Each time you return to the breath, you improve your capacity for focus and presence.

8. Cultivate peace and stillness: As you remain connected to your breath, allow a sense of peace and stillness to permeate your being. Embrace the present moment entirely, surrendering to the rhythm of your breath and the tranquility that comes inside you. Let go of any ideas, worries, or distractions, and simply be with the breath.

9. Practice with regularity: Commit to a regular practice of mindful breathing. Start with a few minutes each day and progressively increase the duration as you get more comfortable. Consistency is crucial to obtaining the benefits of this exercise.

10. Extend Mindful Breathing to Daily Life: As you gain experience with mindful breathing, apply this practice to your daily life. Whether you're engaged in normal activities, encountering problems, or experiencing periods of stress, pause and take a few deliberate breaths. Allow the

serenity and presence acquired through mindful breathing to permeate your daily experiences.

Remember, the beauty of mindful breathing rests in its simplicity. By paying attention to the breath, you tap into a reservoir of tranquility and inner peace that is always accessible to you. Embrace this practice with openness and curiosity, and may it bring you calm and a deeper connection to the present moment.

3.1 Breathe In, Relax Out: Mindful Breathing for Inner Calm

In the fast-paced and demanding world we live in, finding moments of inner stillness and serenity becomes crucial for our well-being. One strong way to foster a sense of calm and tranquility is through attentive breathing. By intentionally focusing on our breath, we can tap into a profound source of inner tranquility. Let's study the practice of mindful breathing for inner calm in greater detail:

1. Find a peaceful location. Begin by finding a peaceful and comfortable location where you can sit or lie down without distractions. Create a setting that encourages a sense of calm and tranquility, allowing you to completely engage in the practice.

2. Settle into a Comfortable Position: Choose a comfortable position that helps you feel relaxed and at ease. You can sit on a cushion or chair or lie down on a comfy surface. Ensure that your body is supported and that you can keep an open posture.

3. Direct Your Awareness to Your Breath: Close your eyes or soften your focus, and direct your attention to your breath. Notice the natural flow of your breath as it enters and departs your body. Be conscious of the sensation of the breath in your nostrils or the rising and falling of your abdomen.

. Breathe in: Take a slow and deep breath in through your nose, allowing the air to fill your lungs. Notice the sensation of the breath entering your body. Feel your chest and abdomen slowly expand as you inhale, bringing a sense of sustenance and energy.

5. Relax Out: As you exhale, let the breath flow slowly and deeply through your nose or mouth. Allow your body to soften and let go of any tension or stress. Feel a sense of comfort and relaxation as you exhale, letting go of any worries or fears.

6. Focus on the Breath: Direct your focus to the complete breath cycle, from the inhale to the exhale. Follow the breath with your consciousness, observing its flow and rhythm. Stay present with each breath, gently and non-judgmentally drawing your attention back whenever it wanders.

7. Embrace the Present Moment: Let go of any distractions or ideas about the past or future. Fully embrace the present moment by anchoring your awareness in the sensations of your breath. Allow yourself to thoroughly enjoy each breath, savoring the sensation of tranquility and relaxation it gives.

8. Cultivate Inner Peace: As you continue to practice mindful breathing, observe how it cultivates a sense of inner peace inside you. With each inhalation, invite a sense of serenity and tranquility into your being. With each exhalation, let go of any tension, stress, or restlessness. Allow the breath to bring you into a state of deep relaxation and calm.

9. Stay with the Breath: Maintain your focus on the breath for a few minutes or as long as it feels comfortable for you. As ideas or distractions occur, notice them without judgment and gently return your focus back to the breath. Cultivate a sense of patience and gentleness with oneself during the practice.

10. Carry Inner Calm into Daily Life: As you end your mindful breathing practice, carry the experience of inner calm with you into your daily life. Whenever you feel anxious, overwhelmed, or in need of grounding, take a moment to reconnect with your breath. Use mindful breathing as a way to find inner quiet and restore a sense of balance amidst life's hardships.

By incorporating mindful breathing into your daily routine, you can tap into a deep well of inner calm and peace. Remember, the practice is simple yet profound. Embrace each breath as an opportunity to relax, let go, and cultivate serenity within yourself. May your journey of mindful breathing bring you a lasting sense of

3.2 Cultivating Balance: Unlocking the Secrets of Mindful Breathing

Mindful breathing is a wonderful skill that allows you to build equilibrium in your life. By turning your attention to the breath and cultivating awareness, you can unlock the mysteries of mindful breathing and bring harmony to your mind, body, and soul. Let's investigate how attentive breathing might help you cultivate balance:

1. Centering Yourself: Mindful breathing serves as an anchor that helps you center yourself in the present moment. When you focus on your breath, you take your attention away from past regrets or future fears and center yourself in the here and now. This brings a sense of equilibrium by allowing you to let go of distractions and connect with your inner self.

2. Regulating Emotions: Our breath is intricately linked to our emotions. When we encounter stress, worry, or overwhelm, our respiration tends

to become shallow and fast. By practicing mindful breathing, you may actively slow down and deepen your breath, stimulating the body's relaxation response and relaxing the nervous system. This management of the breath has a direct impact on balancing and harmonizing your emotional state.

3. Cultivating Awareness: Mindful breathing cultivates a heightened sense of awareness. As you notice each inhale and expiration, you gain a better awareness of your body, mind, and emotions. This awareness allows you to notice imbalances or areas of strain, both physically and psychologically, and take action to resolve them. Through this process, you acquire insight into yourself, developing a stronger sense of balance and well-being.

4. Enhancing Mental Clarity: When the mind is fragmented or overburdened, it can be tough to establish equilibrium. Mindful breathing soothes the mind and brings clarity to your thoughts. By focusing on the breath, you create room for mental calm and quietude, allowing you to approach situations with better clarity and make judgments from a place of balance and wisdom.

5. Developing Resilience: Life is filled with ups and downs, and establishing balance is vital for navigating these changes. Mindful breathing helps you develop resilience by teaching you to stay present and grounded during tough moments. Through the practice, you create

an inner steadiness that helps you respond to adversities with equanimity, adaptability, and grace.

6. Connecting Mind, Body, and Spirit: Mindful breathing promotes a deep connection between your mind, body, and spirit. As you focus your attention on the breath, you unify these components of your existence, producing a harmonic unification. This connection gives a sense of wholeness and balance, uniting you with your genuine self and fostering overall well-being.

7. Nurturing Self-Care: Taking time for mindful breathing is an act of self-care. It is a gentle reminder to slow down, be present, and prioritize your well-being. By adopting regular mindful breathing activities into your daily routine, you commit to nourishing yourself and fostering harmony in all areas of your life.

8. Creating Space for Stillness: In the fast-paced world we live in, stillness is a vital gift that allows us to achieve balance. Mindful breathing creates a sacred space for calm within you. As you focus on your breath, you encourage periods of calm and quiet, creating a haven from the activity and confusion of ordinary life. This calm rejuvenates and heals, allowing you to approach life with a stronger sense of balance.

9. Expanding Compassion: Mindful breathing opens the door to compassion, both for yourself and others. As you create equilibrium

within, you gain a deep sense of empathy and understanding. This compassion spreads beyond yourself, producing harmonious relationships and a compassionate presence in the world.

3.3 Techniques and Practices for Mindful Breathing Bliss

Mindful breathing is a gateway to tranquility and inner peace. By combining certain techniques and practices into your mindful breathing regimen, you can intensify your experience and reach a higher level of happiness. Here are some tools and activities to help your mindful breathing journey:

1. Deep Belly Breathing: Begin by focusing on deep belly breathing, also known as diaphragmatic breathing. Place one hand on your abdomen and the other on your chest. As you inhale, allow your belly to expand, filling it with air. Feel the rising of your abdomen, and as you exhale, let your belly softly sink. Deep belly breathing promotes relaxation, oxygenates the body, and amplifies the calming benefits of mindful breathing.

2. Counting the Breath: Another way to increase mindful breathing is to count your breaths. After each exhalation, silently count "one" in your mind. With the following exhalation, count "two" and continue up to a

count of ten. Then start over from scratch. This counting helps anchor your attention on the breath and cultivates a focused mind.

3. Stretching the Breath: Experiment with stretching your breath to intensify the relaxation response. Slowly prolong the duration of your inhalations and exhalations, making them smooth and gentle. You can try breathing for a count of four, holding the breath for a count of four, and then exhaling for a count of four. Adjust the count based on what seems comfortable for you. Lengthening the breath creates a mood of relaxation and tranquility.

4. Visualization: Incorporate visualization techniques into your mindful breathing practice. As you inhale, envision taking in pleasant, tranquil energy or breathing in a soothing color or light. With each breath, visualize removing any tension, stress, or negativity from your body and mind. Visualization enhances the mind-body link and intensifies the experience of tranquility and happiness.

5. Mindful Body Scan: Combine mindful breathing with a body scan approach. As you inhale, direct your consciousness to a specific portion of your body, and as you exhale, release any tension or tightness in that location. Gradually move your focus throughout your body, bringing mindfulness and calm to each part. The combination of attentive breathing and body scanning intensifies the sense of tranquility and promotes general well-being.

6. Loving-Kindness Meditation: Integrate loving-kindness meditation with mindful breathing to create a sense of compassion and goodwill towards yourself and others. As you breathe in, silently chant lines such as "May I be happy, may I be peaceful, and may I be filled with love."

With each breath, extend these desires to others, starting with loved ones, then neutral folks, and even those you may find challenging. Combining mindful breathing with loving-kindness meditation improves your capacity for kindness and develops a deep sense of connection and joy.

7. Incorporating natural sounds or music: Enhance the delightful experience of mindful breathing by incorporating soothing natural sounds or quiet instrumental music. You can choose sounds like ocean waves, birdsong, or calm musical tunes that resonate with you. These noises create a quiet ambiance, enhancing your relaxation and encouraging a serene state of mind.

8. Mindful Walking: Take your mindful breathing practice beyond sitting meditation by adding it to mindful walking. Find a pleasant outdoor setting or a quiet interior room where you can walk slowly and thoughtfully. As you walk, synchronize your breath with your steps, paying attention to the sensation of each inhale and expiration.

Notice the contact of your feet with the ground, the movement of your body, and the surrounding environment. Mindful walking blends the advantages of physical movement with the peacefulness of mindful breathing, offering a balanced way to grow blissful and present.

9. Breath Awareness in Regular Life: Extend the practice of mindful breathing into your regular activities. Throughout the day, pause and focus your attention on your breath, even during ordinary duties like washing dishes, commuting, or waiting in line.

By bringing breath awareness into your daily life, you infuse each moment with calm and mindfulness, producing a sense of tranquility despite the rush of daily tasks.

10. Gratitude and Reflection: At the end of your mindful breathing exercise, take a moment to express gratitude for the opportunity to create calm and inner peace. Reflect on the results of the practice, recognizing any beneficial shifts in your well-being, clarity of thought, or general sense of tranquility. Embrace a sense of thankfulness for your breath, the source of life and vitality within you.

11. Consistency and Patience: Remember that the road to mastering calm through mindful breathing is a continuous one. Be patient with yourself and maintain consistency in your practice. Set aside dedicated time each day to grow your mindfulness and breath awareness. Over time, you will establish a deeper connection with your breath, revealing a wellspring of serenity that you may draw from in any situation.

12. Seek Guidance and Support: If you feel the need for extra guidance and support in your mindful breathing journey, try receiving instruction from a meditation teacher or joining a mindfulness group or class. Connecting with like-minded folks and learning from experienced practitioners can increase your understanding and provide vital ideas to strengthen your practice.

By accepting these approaches and practices for mindful breathing happiness, you open yourself to a world of tranquility, inner peace, and presence. Embrace the simplicity and power of mindful breathing as you traverse life's ups and downs, and may it become a profound source of peace and well-being in your daily life.

Chapter 4

Guided Imagery: A Journey to Inner Peace

In the pursuit of inner peace, guided imagery is a powerful technique that can transport you to a world of tranquility and deep relaxation. By using your imagination, guided imagery allows you to create vivid mental images that evoke a sense of calm and harmony within. In this chapter, we will explore the technique of guided imagery and its power to guide you on a journey to inner calm.

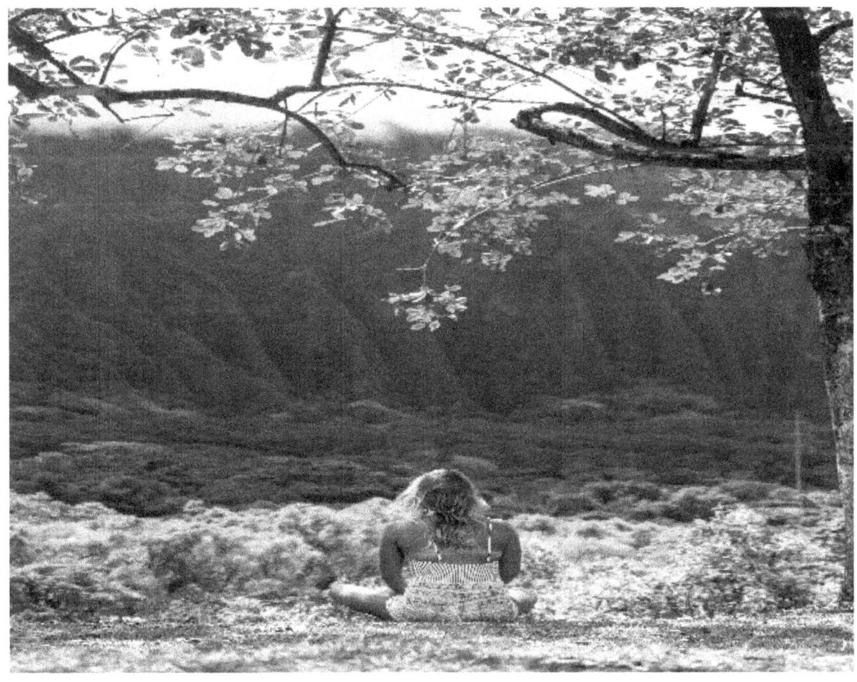

4.1 Guided Imagery: Gateway to a Serene Mind

In the quest for inner peace and tranquility, guided imagery acts as a strong tool to unlock the door to a quiet mind. Guided imaging involves employing vivid mental imagery to generate a sensory experience in the mind, guiding the imagination to inspire a sensation of tranquility, relaxation, and inner harmony. This exercise helps you explore the depths of your imagination and tap into the healing power of your mind. Here, we dig into the world of guided imagery and its potential to transport you on a journey towards inner calm.

1. Understanding Guided Imagery: Guided imagery includes engaging your senses and imagination to create a mental landscape or scenario that supports relaxation and tranquility. It is a style of meditation that uses visualization techniques to produce happy and relaxing experiences. Through the power of visualization, you can achieve profound levels of peace and serenity within yourself.

2. Creating a Safe Area: Begin by choosing a peaceful and comfortable area where you may relax without interruptions. Sit or lie down in a comfortable position, ensuring that your body feels at ease. Take a few deep breaths to quiet your thoughts and release any stress.

3. Guided Imagery Script: To begin your guided imagery practice, you may either write your own visualization script or choose pre-recorded guided imagery sessions available online or through meditation applications. The screenplay often walks you through a serene setting, describing the sensory elements and asking you to immerse yourself in the experience.

4. Engaging the Senses: As the guided imagery unfolds, engage your senses in the visualization. Imagine the sights, sounds, smells, tastes, and textures of the scenario being described. Allow your thoughts to vividly depict each detail, making the experience as real as possible. By fully immersing yourself in the sensory parts of your vision, you increase your connection to the serene images.

5. Deepening Relaxation: Guided imagery often incorporates relaxation techniques such as deep breathing and progressive muscle relaxation. The script may invite you to focus on your breath, guiding you to take slow, deep breaths that promote relaxation and a sense of ease. It may also prompt you to scan your body for any areas of tension and consciously release that tension as you progress through the imagery.

6. Exploring Inner Landscapes: Guided imagery can take you on a journey through various landscapes, such as a serene beach, a lush forest, or a peaceful garden. Allow yourself to fully immerse in the mental imagery, exploring the details and sensations of each scene. Let your imagination guide you as you walk along the beach, feel the warmth of the sun on your skin, or listen to the

gentle lapping of waves. Through this exploration, you create a space within your mind that cultivates serenity and tranquility.

7. Embracing Emotional Healing: Guided imagery can also be a tool for emotional healing and release. As you engage in the visualization, notice any emotions that arise. Allow yourself to fully experience and acknowledge these emotions without judgment. Visualize them gently dissipating, replaced by a sense of calmness and inner peace. The guided imagery session can provide a safe space for emotional healing and offer a pathway to cultivate greater emotional well-being.

8. Gradual Progression: Guided imagery can be practiced at varied lengths, ranging from a few minutes to lengthy sessions. Begin with shorter sessions and progressively increase the duration as you get more comfortable. Consistency in your practice will deepen your connection to the imagery and increase its transforming benefits.

4.2 Unlocking Your Imagination: The Magic of Guided Imagery

Guided imagery is a powerful technique that harnesses the imagination to produce vivid mental images and experiences, guiding us on a journey to inner calm. By engaging our senses and using the creative potential of our thoughts, guided imagery can take us to quiet landscapes, healing surroundings, and inner realms of tranquility. In this section, we examine the wonder of guided imagery and how it can unlock the full capacity of our imagination for inner calm.

1. The Power of Imagination: Our imagination is a gateway to endless possibilities. It permits us to transcend the constraints of our physical reality and delve into the immensity of our inner universe. Through guided imagery, we can harness the transforming power of our imagination to create and explore tranquil, harmonious landscapes within our thoughts.

2. Creating the Ideal Setting: Guided imagery begins by creating a safe and calm setting in your mind. Close your eyes and take a few deep breaths to calm your body and mind. Visualize a peaceful environment that resonates with you—whether it's a remote beach, a serene forest, or a soothing garden. Engage your senses to make the imagery vivid and genuine. Notice the colors, textures, scents, and sounds of this wonderful atmosphere, immersing yourself in its calm.

3. Guided Imagery Scripts: Guided imagery frequently entails following a script or listening to a tape that guides you through a certain visualization. These scripts can be obtained from books, meditation applications, or guided imagery recordings. The screenplay will take you on a journey, explaining the sights, sounds, and experiences you meet

along the way. Allow yourself to totally immerse yourself in the experience, submitting to the guidance and allowing your imagination to paint the surroundings.

4. Engaging the Senses: The brilliance of guided imagery rests in the ability to engage all of your senses. As you picture a serene scene, bring it to life by noticing the nuances. Imagine the gentle caress of a wind on your skin, the aroma of flowers in the air, the warmth of the sun on your face, the sound of leaves rustling, and the sensation of soft grass beneath your feet. By activating all your senses, you improve the reality of the imagery and deepen your experience of inner serenity.

5. Embodying Peaceful States: During guided imagery, you can also nurture specific emotions and states of mind that promote inner calm. Imagine yourself enveloped by a golden radiance of calmness and serenity. Visualize the release of stress and concerns, allowing a deep sense of relaxation to sweep over you. Embrace feelings of gratitude, love, and compassion, creating a condition of inner harmony and contentment. Allow these emotions to pervade your being, producing a profound sense of tranquility.

6. Personalizing Your Imagery: Guided imagery can be modified to meet your preferences and needs. Feel free to change the scripts or build your own visualizations that resonate with you. Explore diverse settings, places, and circumstances that generate a sense of inner tranquility

within you. Your creativity is infinite, and by changing the imagery, you can open a deeper connection to your inner self and boost the transforming impact of the practice.

7. Integration and Reflection: After the guided imagery session, spend a few moments integrating the experience. Slowly bring your consciousness back to the present, wriggling your fingers and toes. Reflect on the imagery and the emotions it evoked.

4.3 Enhancing Relaxation with Guided Imagery Techniques

Guided imagery is a strong practice that can deepen your relaxation and produce a profound sensation of inner peace. By employing visualization and imagination, you can tap into the power of your mind to produce relaxing images, sensations, and emotions. Here are some strategies to increase relaxation with guided imagery:

1. Creating a Peaceful Setting: Begin by finding a peaceful and comfortable location where you may rest without distractions. Close your eyes and envision yourself in a tranquil and serene place of your choice. It may be a lovely beach, a calm woodland, or a comfortable lodge near a lake.

Visualize the nuances of this setting, engaging all your senses. Imagine the sights, sounds, fragrances, and even textures you would encounter in this tranquil atmosphere. Allow yourself to totally absorb the experience, feeling a deep sensation of relaxation and peace.

2. Progressive Muscle Relaxation: Combine guided imagery with progressive muscle relaxation to increase relaxation throughout your body. Begin by envisioning a wave of serenity going through your body from head to toe. As you visualize this wave, focus on each muscle group, starting from your brow and progressing lower. Visualize each muscle group becoming progressively more-calm and at ease as the wave travels through. This combination of visualization and muscular relaxation creates deep physical and mental calm.

3. Safe sanctuary Visualization: Imagine a safe sanctuary where you can retreat in times of stress or discomfort. This can be a serene refuge within your imagination, a place that provides you with a great sense of security and tranquility. Visualize the details of this haven, such as comfortable surroundings, soothing colors, and objects that generate a sense of tranquility. Whenever you feel overwhelmed, you can mentally visit this safe haven, allowing its calming power to wash over you, offering consolation and tranquility.

4. Nature Immersion: Guided imagery can bring you into the embrace of nature, increasing your relaxation. Visualize yourself surrounded by the

beauty of nature, whether it's standing beneath a spectacular waterfall, walking through a sun-dappled forest, or lying on a grassy meadow under a clear blue sky. Engage your senses, envisioning the gentle wind, the aroma of flowers, the warmth of the sunlight on your skin, and the soothing sounds of nature. Allow the therapeutic power of nature to nurture your spirit and boost your relaxation.

5. Emotional Release and Healing: Guided imagery can also aid emotional release and healing. Visualize a quiet brook or river flowing nearby, symbolizing the flow of your emotions. As you breathe deeply and relax, imagine any negative feelings or stress being carried away by the stream, leaving you feeling lighter and more at peace. Visualize healing light or warmth entering your body, easing any emotional wounds and restoring a sense of emotional well-being. This exercise can be particularly helpful during times of stress, sadness, or anxiety.

6. Guided Visualization Recordings: Utilize guided visualization recordings to boost your relaxation practice. There are several guided imagery resources accessible, including audio recordings, applications, and internet platforms. These recordings offer professionally guided visualizations that can bring you through a range of relaxation journeys, providing structure and support for your practice. Choose recordings that resonate with you and explore different topics or settings to find what provides you with the deepest sense of relaxation.

7. Color Visualization: Explore the relaxing influence of colors through guided imagery. Close your eyes and envision a specific color that provides you with a sensation of tranquility, such as soothing blue or tranquil green. Visualize this color covering your entire body, infusing you with a deep sensation of serenity and contentment. Allow the hue to wash away any tension or stress, replacing it with a profound sense of peace and serenity.8. Inner Sanctuary Visualization: Create a personal inner sanctuary within your thoughts where you may retire whenever you need a moment of relaxation and refreshment. Visualize this sanctuary as a space that embodies your inner calm and well-being. It might be a pleasant room, a quiet garden, or any other area that resonates with you. Fill this sanctuary with aspects that provide you comfort, such as soft lighting, comfortable furniture, or relaxing smells. Whenever you enter your inner sanctuary, allow yourself to fully immerse yourself in its tranquility, letting go of any outward anxieties or concerns.

9. Guided Journey Visualization: Embark on a guided journey visualization that takes you on a tranquil and pleasant adventure within your imagination. This could involve envisioning yourself floating on a tranquil river, flying through the clouds, or exploring a gorgeous area. Allow your thoughts to take you through this adventure, experiencing the sights, sounds, and sensations along the way. Embrace the sense of liberation and relaxation that comes with this guided imagery, letting go of any mental or emotional burdens.

10. Self-Healing Visualization: Use guided imagery as a method for self-healing and rejuvenation. Visualize healing energy or light entering your body, flowing through every cell, and renewing your complete being. Imagine this energy mending and correcting any places of stress, discomfort, or imbalance inside you. Allow yourself to embrace this healing energy fully, embracing the restoration and regeneration it gives to your body, mind, and spirit.

11. Guided Affirmations: Combine guided imagery with affirmations to increase relaxation and cultivate positive ideas and feelings. Choose affirmations that resonate with you and encourage your desired state of relaxation and peace. As you engage in guided imagery, silently repeat these affirmations to yourself, incorporating them into the visions and feelings you are experiencing. This combination stimulates pleasant thoughts and feelings, deepening your relaxation and producing a sense of inner harmony.

12. Personalized Guided Imagery: Tailor your guided imagery practice to suit your particular tastes and needs. Experiment with generating your own guided visualizations depending on what brings you calm and peace. You can write down scripts or simply speak them out during your practice. Personalized guided imagery allows you to connect with your particular imagery and experiences, making the relaxing process much more meaningful and beneficial for you.

As you add these guided imagery techniques to your relaxation practice, remember to approach them with an open and fun perspective. Allow your imagination to take you on a journey of inner peace and tranquility. Embrace the transformational power of guided imagery as it feeds your mind, body, and spirit, offering you deeper relaxation and a refreshed sense of well-being.

Chapter 5

Progressive Muscle Relaxation: Unwind and Let Go

Progressive Muscle Relaxation (PMR) is a technique that induces profound relaxation by repeatedly tensing and releasing different muscle groups in the body. It is an efficient way of unwinding and letting go of bodily and mental strain. In this chapter, we will study the practice of PMR and its benefits for creating a state of deep relaxation and tranquility.

Progressive muscle calm includes consciously tensing and then relaxing different muscle groups to achieve a deep sense of calm. The practice helps enhance body awareness and teaches you to detect the difference between tension and relaxation in various parts of your body. By actively releasing tension, you can lessen muscle tightness, relieve stress, and foster a feeling of serenity.

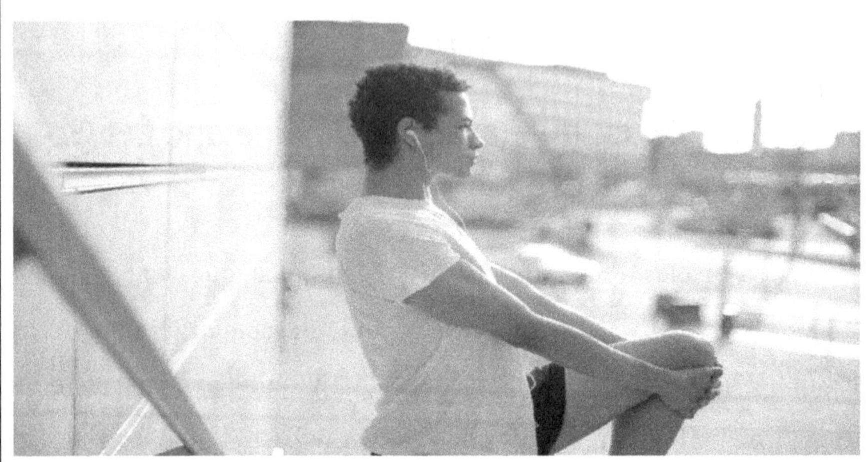

5.1 Melt Away Tension: The Power of Progressive Muscle Relaxation

Progressive muscle relaxation is a technique that allows you to reduce tension and achieve profound relaxation throughout your body. By systematically tensing and then releasing different muscle groups, you can build a profound sensation of comfort and tranquility. Here's an exploration of the power of progressive muscle relaxation:

Understanding Progressive Muscle Relaxation: Progressive muscle relaxation requires purposefully tensing and then releasing specific muscle groups, one at a time, in a methodical manner. By purposefully tensing the muscles and then letting go, you develop your awareness of tension and learn to relax profoundly. This technique is founded on the premise that the body and mind are interrelated, and by reducing physical tension, you can also encourage mental and emotional relaxation.

The Benefits of Progressive Muscle Relaxation:

1. Physical Relaxation: Progressive muscular relaxation allows you to recognize and release muscle tension, generating a feeling of physical calm. As you practice consistently, you may feel a reduction in muscular pain, stiffness, and discomfort, boosting your overall physical well-being.

2. Stress Reduction: Tension typically accumulates in the body due to stress and anxiety. Progressive muscle relaxation helps to reduce this tension, lowering the physiological and psychological consequences of stress. It activates the body's relaxation response, resulting in a calmer and more serene state of mind

. Improved Sleep: By actively releasing muscle tension before bedtime, gradual muscle relaxation can boost the quality of your sleep. As your body and mind relax, you may have a more peaceful and refreshing sleep, awakening refreshed and energetic.

4. Emotional Balance: The reduction of physical tension through progressive muscle relaxation can also help with emotional balance. As

you let go of muscular tension, you may experience a sense of peace, less irritation, and an increased capacity to handle emotions efficiently.

The Process of Progressive Muscle Relaxation: To achieve progressive muscle relaxation, follow these steps:

1. Find a quiet and comfortable area where you can relax without distractions. Sit or lie down in a relaxed position.

2. Begin by taking a few deep breaths, allowing your body and mind to calm.

3. Start with a specific muscle group, such as your hands or feet. Tense the muscles in that area by clenching or squeezing them for around 5–10 seconds.
4. Release the tension in that muscle group immediately and completely, enabling the muscles to relax completely. Focus on the sensation of relaxation as the tension fades away.

5. Take a few moments to observe and enjoy the sensation of relaxation in that muscle group before moving on to the next one.

6. Repeat this method with different muscle groups throughout your body, working your way up or down progressively. Common muscle groups to include are the hands, arms, shoulders, neck, face, abdomen, buttocks, legs, and feet.

7. As you proceed through each muscle group, continue to focus on the contrast between tension and relaxation, experiencing the developing sense of tranquility.

8. Once you have gone over all the muscle groups, take a few minutes to simply appreciate the general feeling of relaxation throughout your body.

9. When you're ready, slowly bring your consciousness back to the present moment. Gently stretch and move your body, allowing yourself to adjust back to your typical routines.

Remember, the key to gradual muscle relaxation is to approach it with a gentle and non-judgmental attitude. Each session is an opportunity to let go of tension and encourage relaxation. As you practice regularly, you may discover that your body gets more attuned to stress and is better able to release it, resulting in a greater A Step-by-Step Guide to Progressive Muscle Relaxation

5.2: A Step-by-Step Guide to Progressive Muscle Relaxation

Progressive Muscle Relaxation (PMR) is a technique that involves systematically tensing and releasing muscle groups to produce deep relaxation and release physical tension. By actively focusing on different parts of the body, you can become more aware of tension and learn to let go. Here is a step-by-step approach to practicing progressive muscle relaxation:

1. Find a quiet and comfortable area where you can relax without distractions. Sit or lie down in a position that allows you to fully relax your body.

2. Close your eyes and take a few deep breaths to quiet your thoughts and bring your attention to the present moment.

3. Begin by focusing on your breathing. Take a slow, deep breath through your nose, filling your lungs with air. Hold your breath for a time, and then gently exhale through your mouth, releasing any tension or stress with each breath.

4. Start with your feet. Bring your attention to your toes and softly curl them, tensing the muscles in your feet. Hold this tension for a few seconds, and then release it entirely, allowing your feet to relax totally.

5. Gradually work your way up through your body, progressing to your calves and thighs. Tense the muscles in each place for a few seconds and then release them, feeling the tension melt away. Pay attention to the sensations of tension and relaxation as you travel through each muscle

group.

6. Continue to your buttocks and pelvic area, tensing the muscles in that region and then releasing the tension. Move up to your abdomen, tensing the muscles there and then letting go fully.

7. Move to your hands, creating a fist and gripping the muscles forcefully. Hold for a few seconds, and then release, allowing your hands to soften and relax.

8. Proceed to your arms and shoulders, paying attention to the muscles in those places. Tense the muscles by raising your shoulders towards your ears, hold for a few seconds, and then release, feeling the tension disappear.

9. Move up to your neck, tensing the muscles by slowly tilting your head back and experiencing the stretch. Hold for a second, and then release, allowing your neck to relax and return to its normal position.

10. Finally, focus on your face and head. Scrunch up your face, tensing all the muscles, and then release, letting go of any tension in your facial muscles. Feel your forehead, eyes, jaw, and all the little muscles in your face relax.

11. Take a few moments to scan your body and detect any leftover places of tension. If you locate any, turn your attention to those locations and

actively release the tension, allowing your entire body to enter a state of deep relaxation.

12. Take a few more deep breaths, experiencing the relaxation spreading throughout your body with each exhale. Enjoy the sensations of calmness and serenity that occur from this practice.

13. When you are ready, softly open your eyes and bring your consciousness back to the present moment. Take a moment to appreciate the calm and peacefulness you have cultivated through progressive muscle calm.

Practice progressive muscle relaxation consistently to become more aware of the sensations of tension and relaxation in your body. With time, you will develop a better awareness of where stress tends to gather and be able to actively release it, promoting a sense of deep relaxation and well-being.

5.3 Rejuvenate Your Body and Mind with Progressive Muscle Relaxation

Progressive Muscle Relaxation (PMR) is a technique that promotes deep relaxation by progressively tensing and then releasing different muscle groups in your body. By partaking in this exercise, you may relieve tension, reduce stress, and refresh both your body and mind. Here's how you can refresh yourself using Progressive Muscle Relaxation:

1. Find a peaceful area: Begin by locating a peaceful and comfortable area where you may fully focus on the practice without interruptions. It could be a serene room, a pleasant area of your home, or someplace that creates a sense of tranquility.

2. Assume a Comfortable Position: Sit or lie down in a comfortable position, allowing your body to totally relax. Close your eyes and take a few deep breaths to center yourself and bring your attention to the present moment.

3. Systematically Tense and Relax: Begin the Progressive Muscle Relaxation practice by focusing on individual muscle groups one at a time. Start with your toes and work your way up through your body, progressively tensing and then releasing each muscle group. For example, you can start by curling your toes tightly for a few seconds, and then release them, letting the tension to flow away. Move on to your feet, calves, thighs, and so on, until you reach your face and head.

4. Focus on the Sensation: As you tense each muscle group, pay attention to the sensation of tension and stiffness. Notice how it feels to retain the tension in that region. Then, when you remove the tension, examine the opposing sense

of relaxation and the relief that comes with it. Stay present and conscious during the procedure, focusing on the feelings in each muscle group.

5. Use Breath Awareness: Incorporate deep, slow breaths into your practice to increase relaxation. As you tense a muscle group, take a deep breath in, and as you release the tension, exhale gently, letting rid of any leftover tension in that place. Allow your breath to be a guiding force, helping you reduce tension and deepen relaxation with each exhalation.

6. Progress at Your Own Pace: Progress through each muscle group at a pace that feels comfortable for you. Take your time to completely experience and release the tension in each place before going on to the next. Remember, the purpose is not to rush but to foster deep relaxation and renewal.

7. Notice the Contrast: As you proceed through the practice, pay notice to the contrast between tension and relaxation. Appreciate the difference in sensation and the sense of relief that comes with releasing tension from each muscle group. Embrace the feeling of lightness and ease that comes when your body relaxes.

8. Embrace Full-Body Relaxation: After moving through each muscle area, take a minute to appreciate the overall sense of relaxation and rejuvenation that you've fostered throughout your body. Allow yourself to totally engage in the

sensation of relaxation from head to toe, feeling a sense of peace and regeneration spreading throughout your entire being.

9. Practice Regularly: To enjoy the full advantages of Progressive Muscle Relaxation, make it a regular component of your self-care regimen. Set aside committed time each day or week to engage in this activity. The more you practice, the more adept you will become at releasing tension and revitalizing your body and mind.

10. Extend Relaxation Beyond the Practice: As you become comfortable with the method of Progressive Muscle Relaxation, attempt to carry the relaxation techniques into your daily life. Use the abilities you've learned to detect and release tension in specific muscle groups when you encounter stress or discomfort

Chapter 6

Sleep Hygiene: Creating a Restful Environment

Creating a tranquil environment is vital for getting adequate sleep and promoting overall well-being. Your sleep sanctuary should be a refuge of peace and comfort, designed to assist relaxation and ensure a deep and restful rest.

By practicing sleep hygiene habits and taking intentional measures to build your sleep environment, you may create the optimum conditions for a comfortable night's sleep. From tidying and organizing your home to maximizing lighting, choosing comfortable bedding, and avoiding noise, each factor plays a key role in establishing a tranquil mood.

Additionally, introducing calming colors, managing temperature and air quality, developing a nighttime routine, and decreasing the presence of devices all contribute to the construction of a sleep sanctuary that promotes peace and rejuvenation. By spending time and effort into planning your sleep environment, you may optimize your sleep quality, improve your overall sleep hygiene, and experience the profound advantages of restful and restorative sleep.

6.1 Crafting Your Sleep Sanctuary: The Importance of Sleep Hygiene

Creating a tranquil environment is vital for supporting excellent sleep and providing adequate rest and regeneration. Your sleep sanctuary, the location where you sleep, plays a significant part in establishing healthy sleep patterns and increasing the overall quality of your sleep. Here are some crucial factors of sleep hygiene to consider when constructing your sleep sanctuary:

1. comfy Bed and Bedding: Start by ensuring that your bed is comfy and supportive. Choose a mattress and pillows that provide the perfect level of firmness and support for your body. Your bedding should be clean, soft, and inviting. Invest in high-quality linens and blankets that offer a pleasant and comfortable sleep experience.

2. Declutter and Organize: Keep your sleep environment clean, decluttered, and free from distractions. Clutter can produce a sense of disorder and unrest, making it harder to relax and unwind. Remove any unneeded belongings from your bedroom, producing a serene and peaceful space conducive to sleep.

3. Ambient Lighting: Optimize your sleep environment with adequate lighting. Use gentle, pleasant lighting in the evening to create a peaceful ambiance. Avoid bright and harsh lights, as they can interrupt your natural sleep-wake cycle. Consider using blackout curtains or an eye mask to block out exterior light sources that may interfere with your sleep.

4. Noise Control: Minimize noise disruptions that can impair your sleep. If you live in a noisy environment, try earplugs or a white noise machine

to block out undesirable sounds. Alternatively, you can employ soothing sounds like nature noises or calming music to create a serene aural environment that promotes relaxation and sleep.

5. Temperature and ventilation: Keep your sleep environment at a suitable temperature. The ideal room temperature for sleep differs for each individual, but usually, a little cooler atmosphere encourages greater sleep. Ensure sufficient ventilation and airflow in your bedroom, as fresh air can contribute to a more pleasant sleep experience.

6. Technology-Free Zone: Create a technology-free zone in your sleep sanctuary. Electronic devices generate blue light, which can interfere with your body's generation of melatonin, a hormone that governs sleep. Keep electronics such as smartphones, tablets, and computers out of the bedroom, or set them on silent mode and out of your immediate reach.

7. Scent and Aromatherapy: Harness the power of scents to create a comfortable sleep environment. Consider utilizing essential oils recognized for their soothing effects, such as lavender or chamomile. Use a diffuser or lightly spray your mattress with a calming perfume before sleep to encourage relaxation and a sense of tranquility.

8. Establish a nighttime ritual: Develop a consistent nighttime ritual that signals to your body and mind that it's time to unwind and prepare for sleep. This practice can include activities such as reading a book,

practicing relaxation techniques, having a warm bath, or listening to peaceful music. Engaging in a routine can help communicate to your body that it's time to transition from wakefulness to sleep.

9. Limit Stimulants: Avoid consuming stimulants close to bedtime since they can interfere with your ability to fall asleep. Caffeine, nicotine, and alcohol can alter your sleep patterns, making it harder to attain restorative sleep. Instead, go for a relaxing herbal tea or warm milk if you require a pre-bedtime beverage.

10. Create a sleep-friendly perspective: cultivate a good and calm perspective around sleep. Approach bedtime with a sense of relaxation and anticipation of restful sleep. Release any concerns or stressors by using relaxation techniques or journaling before bed. Create an intention to prioritize sleep and respect its importance in preserving your overall well-being.

11. Constant Sleep Routine: Establish a constant sleep routine by going to bed and waking up at the same time each day, even on weekends. This helps regulate your body's internal schedule, making it simpler to go to sleep and wake up normally. Stick to your sleep routine as much as possible to maintain a healthy sleep-wake cycle.

12. Reserve the Bedroom for Sleep and Intimacy: Associate your bedroom largely with sleep and intimacy. Avoid indulging in activities

that are mentally stimulating or stressful in bed, such as working or watching TV. By reserving the bedroom for rest and relaxation, you teach your mind to associate the space with sleep, promoting greater sleep quality.

13. Seek Comfort in Bedtime Rituals: Incorporate pleasant bedtime rituals into your routine. This could involve practicing relaxation methods, such as deep breathing or mild stretching, or engaging in a mindfulness practice like meditation. These rituals can help you unwind, release tension, and prepare your body and mind for a pleasant night's sleep.

14. Evaluate and modify your sleep environment. Regularly analyze your sleep environment to find any variables that may be affecting your sleep quality. Adjust the temperature, lighting, noise levels, and other aspects to create an atmosphere that fosters good sleep. Experiment with different pillows, mattresses, or bedding to find what works best for your comfort.

15. Monitor Your Sleep Hygiene Behaviors: Keep track of your sleep hygiene behaviors and their impact on your sleep quality. Notice how different circumstances, such as screen time, caffeine consumption, or exercise, affect your ability to fall asleep and stay asleep. Use this awareness to make educated modifications and emphasize practices that promote healthy sleep.

By applying these sleep hygiene habits and constructing a sleep sanctuary that encourages calm and tranquility, you may create the ideal setting for refreshing sleep. Remember, healthy sleep is a crucial component of overall

well-being, and by emphasizing sleep hygiene, you are nurturing your body and mind for optimal rest and renewal.

6.2 Establishing Healthy Sleep Habits for Optimal Rest and Renewal

Creating a pleasant sleep environment and adopting healthy sleep habits are vital for ensuring deep and rejuvenating sleep. By applying the following techniques, you can optimize your sleep hygiene and enhance your general well-being:

1. Constant Sleep Routine: Set a constant sleep routine by going to bed and waking up at the same time every day, even on weekends. This helps regulate your body's internal clock and promotes a more normal sleep-wake cycle.

2. Create a Soothing Bedroom: Design your bedroom as a tranquil and peaceful sanctuary dedicated to sleep. Keep the room dark, quiet, and at

a comfortable temperature. Consider using blackout curtains, earplugs, or a white noise machine to shut out any exterior disturbances.

3. Comfortable Sleep Environment: Invest in a comfortable mattress, pillows, and bedding that support your body and provide a cozy sleeping surface. Find a pillow that suits your sleeping position and helps preserve appropriate spinal alignment. Experiment with several mattress firmness levels to find the one that suits your comfort preferences.

4. Limit Electronic Devices: Avoid using electronic devices, such as cellphones, tablets, or computers, before bedtime. The blue light emitted by these devices can interrupt your sleep habits by decreasing the generation of melatonin, a hormone that governs sleep.

5. Relaxation Rituals: Establish a calm pre-sleep ritual to indicate to your body and mind that it's time to wind down. Engage in relaxing activities, such as reading a book, having a warm bath, doing easy stretches, or listening to peaceful music. These rituals help put your body into a state of relaxation and prepare you for a good night's sleep.

6. Avoid Stimulants: Limit or avoid ingesting stimulants such as caffeine, nicotine, and alcohol, especially in the evening. These substances can interfere with your ability to fall asleep and stay asleep throughout the night.

7. Exercise regularly: Engage in frequent physical activity during the day, as it promotes better sleep. However, avoid strenuous exercise close to bedtime, as it might raise awareness and make it difficult to fall asleep. Aim to conclude your exercise program at least a few hours before bedtime.

8. Create a Sleep-Friendly Atmosphere: Make your sleep environment conducive to relaxation by keeping it tidy, clutter-free, and free from distractions. Consider utilizing aromatherapy, such as lavender essential oil, to produce a peaceful scent in your bedroom.

9. Manage Stress: Practice stress-management practices, such as mindfulness meditation, deep breathing exercises, or journaling, to help alleviate tension and worry that can interfere with sleep. Create a worry-free zone before bed by addressing any issues earlier in the day and engaging in relaxation exercises to maintain a serene mood.

10. Limit Napping: If you struggle with nocturnal sleep, limit daytime napping or reduce it to brief power naps of 20–30 minutes. Long naps or resting too close to bedtime can alter your sleep schedule.

11. Evaluate Your Sleep Environment: Periodically check your sleep environment for any variables that may be limiting your sleep quality. Consider elements such as noise levels, light exposure, comfort, and

temperature. Make modifications as needed to enhance your sleep environment.

12. Seek professional treatment: If you frequently battle with sleep disorders after practicing good sleep practices, consider obtaining professional treatment from a sleep specialist or healthcare provider. They can examine you and provide appropriate counseling and treatment choices to address any underlying sleep issues or concerns.

By adopting these strategies into your daily routine, you can cultivate healthy sleep habits and create an environment that encourages restful and rejuvenating sleep.

6.3 Enhancing Your Sleep Environment for Ultimate Serenity

The quality of your sleep is largely influenced by your sleep environment. By adjusting your environment for peace and relaxation, you can create a quiet ambiance that promotes deep and regenerative sleep. Here are some strategies for optimizing your sleep environment for utmost serenity:

1. Declutter and simplify: Keep your sleep environment clean and clutter-free. Remove any superfluous objects from your bedroom that may generate visual or mental distractions. Create a place that encourages a sense of relaxation and serenity, allowing your mind to decompress as you prepare for sleep.

2. Comfortable Bedding and Mattress: Invest in high-quality bedding and a comfy mattress that provide appropriate support for your body. Choose pillows and blankets that suit your tastes and offer optimal comfort. The correct bedding and mattress can dramatically boost your sleep quality and overall tranquility.

3. Optimal Room Temperature: Maintain a comfortable room temperature that is beneficial to sleep. The optimal temperature may vary for each individual, but usually, a chilly and slightly ventilated setting promotes better sleep. Experiment with different temperatures to see what works best for you.

4. Control Noise Levels: Minimize noise disturbances in your sleep surroundings to produce a serene setting. Use earplugs, white noise machines, or relaxing natural sounds to cover external noises and induce relaxation. If required, consider using blackout curtains or an eye mask to block out excessive light and create a darker sleeping environment.

5. Relaxing hues and lighting: Choose soft, relaxing hues for your bedroom walls and decor. Pastel tints, earth tones, or chilly colors can produce a tranquil ambience. Use gentle, warm lighting or dimmer switches to create a soothing ambiance before bed. Avoid bright, harsh lights that can interrupt your sleep-wake cycle.

6. Aromatherapy for Relaxation: Consider utilizing essential oils or aromatherapy diffusers to enrich your sleeping surroundings with peaceful scents. Lavender, chamomile, and sandalwood are known for their soothing characteristics and can help generate a peaceful sleep atmosphere. Ensure appropriate ventilation and observe safety standards when utilizing essential oils.

7. Electronic Device-Free Zone: Create a designated electronic device-free zone in your bedroom. Remove electronic gadgets such as smartphones, tablets, and laptops that emit blue light, which might interfere with your sleep habits. Instead, engage in relaxing activities such as reading a book, performing mild stretching, or engaging in relaxation techniques before bed.

8. Establish a nighttime ritual: Develop a consistent nighttime ritual that helps signal to your body and mind that it's time to unwind and prepare for sleep. Engage in soothing activities such as having a warm bath, doing moderate yoga or stretching, listening to quiet music, or reading a

book. Consistency in your habits can help regulate your body's internal clock and boost your sleep quality.

9. Promote a Sense of Tranquility: Personalize your sleep environment with items that generate a sense of tranquility and relaxation. This can be soothing artwork, nature-inspired decorations, or objects that contain sentimental value and provide you with delight. Surrounding yourself with products that encourage a quiet mentality might lead to a more serene sleep environment.

10. Optimize Comfort and Support: Pay attention to the comfort and support of your sleep basics. Use pillows that align with your desired sleep posture and provide appropriate support for your head and neck. Consider using a mattress topper or investing in a mattress that meets your individual comfort demands. Ensuring maximum comfort and support can considerably enhance your sleep experience.

11. Promote darkness and silence: Ensure that your sleep environment is as dark and silent as possible. Use blackout drapes or blinds to shut off external light sources. If you're unable to eliminate all sources of noise, consider using earplugs or a white noise machine to mask undesirable sounds and create a tranquil ambiance.

12. Comfortable Temperature and Ventilation: Create an optimal sleep environment by adjusting the temperature and maintaining appropriate

ventilation. Keep the room cold and well-ventilated, enabling fresh air to flow. Use fans or air conditioning to maintain a suitable temperature that promotes healthy sleep.

13. Establish a technology-free zone: banish technological devices from your sleeping surroundings. The blue light emitted by cellphones, tablets, and laptops can interfere with your sleep quality. Designate your bedroom as a technology-free zone and avoid using electronic gadgets for at least an hour before bed. Instead, indulge in soothing activities that prepare your mind and body for sleep.

14. Soft and Cozy Bedding: Choose bedding that feels soft and cozy to the touch. Opt for high-quality sheets, blankets, and pillowcases manufactured from soft and breathable materials. Experiment with different textures to find what provides you the most comfort and helps you unwind.

15. Scented Candles or Essential Oils: Incorporate relaxing scents into your sleeping surroundings through scented candles or essential oils. Lavender, chamomile, and jasmine are known for their relaxing effects. Use a diffuser or place a few drops of essential oil on a cotton pad near your bed to create a calm and relaxing aroma.

16. Generate a Clutter-Free Space: Clear away any clutter from your sleeping surroundings to generate a sense of peace and spaciousness. A

clutter-free setting encourages a clear and quiet mind, helping you shift into a relaxed mood. Consider organizing your possessions and locating specific storage locations to make your sleeping environment tidy and serene.

17. Comforting evening routines: Establish evening routines that communicate to your body and mind that it's time to unwind and prepare for sleep. This can include things such as reading a book, practicing moderate stretches or relaxation exercises, writing in a gratitude notebook, or sipping a warm cup of herbal tea. Engaging in these comfortable routines before bed will help you relax and shift into a restful mood.

18. Adjust Your Bedtime Routine: Evaluate your existing bedtime routine and make improvements as appropriate. Aim to develop a consistent sleep schedule by going to bed and waking up at the same time each day, especially on weekends. This regularity helps regulate your body's internal clock and promotes greater sleep quality.

19. Assess and Modify Your Sleep Environment: Periodically assess your sleep environment and make appropriate modifications. Pay attention to any elements that may be interfering with your sleep, such as noise, light, or discomfort. Make modifications accordingly to improve your sleep environment for optimum serenity.

20. Prioritize Your Sleep Environment: Understand the value of building a sleep environment that supports your relaxation and well-being. Prioritize the time and effort needed to develop a calm atmosphere that fosters profound relaxation and renewal. By investing in your sleep environment, you are investing in your overall health and happiness.

By applying these tactics to optimize your sleep environment, you can create an optimal setting that promotes deep relaxation, undisturbed sleep, and ultimate serenity. Remember that developing a perfect sleep environment is a personal process, and it may require some trial and error to find what works best for you. Embrace the process and prioritize self-care by cultivating your sleep environment for the best peaceful experience.

Chapter 7

Yoga Nidra: Deep Relaxation and Rejuvenation

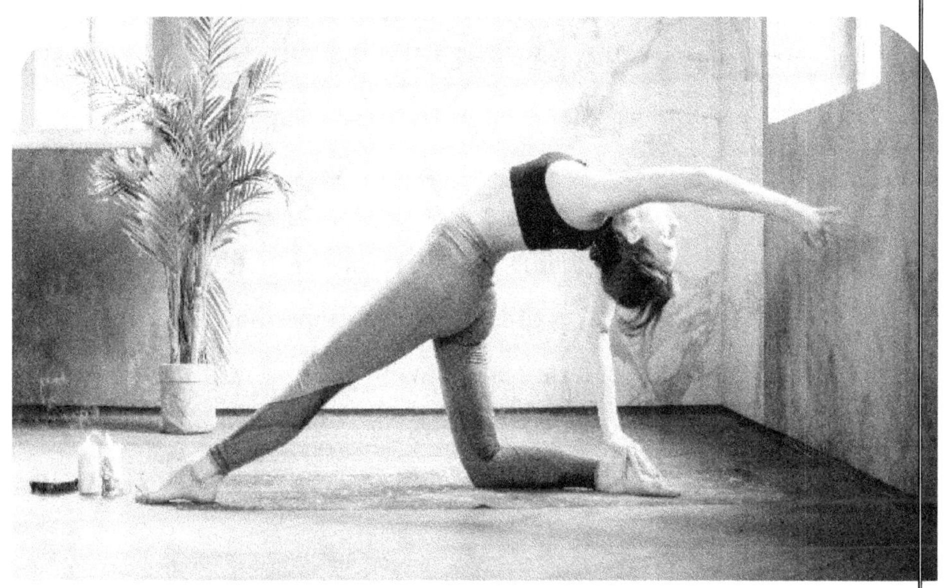

7.1 Yoga Nidra: Embracing Profound Relaxation

Yoga Nidra is a powerful technique that helps you feel profound relaxation, regeneration, and inner serenity. It is also referred to as "yogic sleep" or "psychic sleep" because it creates a condition of conscious sleep where the body and mind are in a state of profound relaxation yet awareness remains awake and alert. By embracing Yoga Nidra, you can tap into the therapeutic potential of profound relaxation. Here's how you can go on this voyage of profound relaxation:

1. Settle into a Comfortable Position: Find a quiet and comfortable location where you can lie down on your back, ensuring that your body is adequately supported. Use props such as blankets, pillows, or an eye cushion to create a pleasant and caring environment. Allow your body to relax totally and yield to the support beneath you.

2. Connect with Your Breath: Begin by taking a few deep breaths, allowing yourself to arrive fully in the present moment. Notice the sensation of the breath entering and leaving your body. Take calm, easy breaths, breathing deeply through your nose and exhaling fully through your mouth. Let each breath quiet your nervous system and put you into a state of relaxation.

3. Set an Intention: Before plunging into the practice of Yoga Nidra, set a clear intention for your session. This can be a basic affirmation or a specific area of your well-being that you wish to focus on during the exercise. By setting an intention, you create a guiding compass for your journey of profound relaxation and restoration.

4. Engage in a Body Scan: Begin to bring your awareness to different regions of your body, starting with your toes and working all the way up

to the top of your head. As you shift your attention to each body part, intentionally release any stress or tightness you may be harboring. Allow the awareness to gradually scan over your body, bringing a sensation of relaxation and ease to each location.

5. Cultivate Witness Consciousness: Throughout the practice of Yoga Nidra, maintain a condition of witness consciousness. Observe the sensations, thoughts, and emotions that arise without judgment or attachment. Allow them to come and go, understanding that you are not defined by them. By nurturing this witness consciousness, you create a space of inner calm and acceptance.

6. Follow the Guided Script: In Yoga Nidra, a guided script is commonly utilized to lead you through the practice. The script may include visions, affirmations, and explicit directions to guide your awareness. Surrender to the guidance of the script, allowing it to carry you deeper into relaxation and restoration.

7. Explore Sensations and Imagery: As you approach a state of profound relaxation, you may experience numerous sensations, visions, or emotions. Embrace these experiences without getting connected to them. Notice the colors, textures, and feelings that arise, letting them flow through your awareness. Trust the wisdom of your subconscious mind as it communicates with you through these sensations and visions.

8. Experience Timelessness: In the state of Yoga Nidra, time loses its traditional meaning. You may discover that times of deep relaxation and silence feel timeless, as if you are floating in a space beyond time and space. Embrace this sensation of timelessness and let go of any impulse to control or influence the passage of time. Allow yourself to fully submit to the moment.

9. Awaken Gradually: Towards the end of your Yoga Nidra practice, you will be guided to gradually return your consciousness back to your physical surroundings. Take your time to reconnect with your body and the external environment. Begin by gently wriggling your fingers and toes, slowly stretching your limbs, and taking a few deep breaths. Take a minute to savor the deep state of relaxation and rejuvenation you have experienced during the practice.

10. Reflect and Integrate: After completing the practice of Yoga Nidra, take a few moments to reflect on your experience. Notice any adjustments or sensations in your body and thoughts. Allow yourself to integrate the benefits of deep relaxation into your daily life. You may opt to journal about your experience, expressing any insights or emotions that have emerged during the practice.

11. Make Yoga Nidra a Regular Practice: To completely enjoy the profound relaxation and renewal of Yoga Nidra, make it a regular component of your self-care regimen. Set aside committed time for this

exercise, whether it's daily or a few times a week. Consistency is crucial to experiencing the cumulative advantages of profound relaxation and inner calm.

12. Investigate Guided Yoga Nidra Resources: If you are new to Yoga Nidra or would need extra guidance, investigate guided Yoga Nidra resources. There are several recordings, apps, and online platforms that offer guided Yoga Nidra sessions given by experienced teachers. Find a resource that connects with you and supports your journey of deep relaxation and restoration.

Yoga Nidra offers a profound road to deep relaxation, regeneration, and inner serenity. By accepting this technique, you can tap into the healing potential of conscious sleep and build a state of profound peace. Allow yourself to fully surrender and experience the peaceful realm of Yoga Nidra as you nurture your body, mind, and spirit.

7.2 Unveiling the Benefits of Yoga Nidra for Sleep and Relaxation

Yoga Nidra, often known as "yogic sleep," is a powerful technique that promotes profound relaxation, regeneration, and restful sleep. It is a guided meditation technique that helps you attain a state of profound relaxation while being cognizant and aware. By adopting Yoga Nidra into your sleep and relaxation practice, you can experience a wide range of advantages. Let's expose some of the primary benefits of practicing Yoga Nidra:

1. Tension Reduction: Yoga Nidra is particularly beneficial for relieving tension and anxiety. As you achieve a state of deep relaxation, it helps quiet your nervous system and stimulates the body's relaxation response. By relieving tension and stress from your mind and body, you can enjoy a better sense of serenity and tranquility.

2. Enhanced Sleep Quality: Yoga Nidra can greatly improve the quality of your sleep. By bringing you into a state of deep relaxation, it helps regulate your sleep-wake cycle and promotes a more comfortable sleep. Regular practice of Yoga Nidra can minimize sleep disruptions and insomnia and promote a deeper and more restful sleep experience.

3. Deep Mind-Body Connection: During a Yoga Nidra session, you build a deep connection between your mind and body. By actively relaxing different sections of your body and bringing awareness to varied feelings, you acquire a heightened sense of self-awareness. This connection strengthens your ability to listen to your body's demands and signals, allowing for improved self-care and overall well-being.

4. Emotional Healing and Balance: Yoga Nidra helps with emotional healing and balance. By accessing deep states of relaxation, you can explore and release repressed emotions, trauma, and bad patterns. It offers a secure and caring space for emotional processing and develops a sense of inner peace, joy, and equanimity.

5. Improved Mental Clarity and Focus: Regular practice of Yoga Nidra promotes mental clarity and focus. By creating a state of profound relaxation, you can lessen mental chatter and quiet the restless mind. This clarity and focus extend beyond the practice itself, enabling you to face daily chores and obstacles with a calmer and more centered perspective.

6. Body-Mind Repair: Yoga Nidra allows for significant physical and mental repair. As you achieve a state of deep relaxation, the body's natural healing processes are stimulated, supporting cellular regeneration, better immunological function, and general physical well-being. It refills your energy levels, leaving you feeling renewed and energized.

7. Cultivation of awareness: Yoga Nidra cultivates awareness, the discipline of being fully present in the present moment. By guiding your attention through diverse sensations, breath awareness, and imagination, it deepens your capacity to be present and alert. This mindfulness pours over into your daily life, producing a stronger sense of clarity, thankfulness, and joy.

8. Self-Discovery and Transformation: Through consistent practice, Yoga Nidra offers a path of self-discovery and personal transformation. As you go into the depths of your being and connect with your inner wisdom, you can acquire insights, clarity, and a better understanding of yourself. This self-awareness and transformation provide the path for personal growth, empowerment, and good change.

7.3: A Step-by-Step Guide to Experiencing the Bliss of Yoga Nidra

Yoga Nidra, also known as yogic sleep, is a potent technique that causes deep relaxation and regeneration. It guides you into a state of profound serenity while being cognizant and aware. Here is a step-by-step guide to experiencing the ecstasy of Yoga Nidra:

1. Find a calm and comfortable area. Begin by finding a calm and tranquil area where you can practice undisturbed. Create a nice atmosphere by employing soft lighting, comfortable cushions, and blankets to support your body during the practice. Lie down on your back in a relaxed position, ensuring that your body is well supported and comfortable.

2. Set an Intention: Take a moment to set a clear intention for your Yoga Nidra practice. This could be anything you intend to grow in or work on, such as profound relaxation, inner peace, self-healing, or releasing tension. Formulate a positive and succinct aim, articulating it silently or aloud with conviction.

3. Relax and center yourself. Close your eyes and take a few deep breaths to relax and center yourself. Allow your body to settle into a state of calm and let go of any tension or tightness. Become aware of the natural rhythm of your breath, focusing on each inhalation and exhalation.

4. Follow the Guided Instructions: Yoga Nidra is often practiced utilizing a guided audio recording or a teacher's voice. Listen to the instructions and follow along, allowing yourself to be guided through the many stages of the practice. The coaching will bring you through a systematic relaxation of different regions of your body and a voyage of imagery and self-awareness.

5. Body Scan and Relaxation: Begin the activity by bringing your attention to different sections of your body. Mentally scan each place, starting from the toes and continuing upward to your legs, body, arms, and head. As you focus on each body area, intentionally release any tension or tightness, allowing the muscles to relax and soften.

6. Explore Sensations and Breath Awareness: As you proceed through the practice, you may be led to bring awareness to other sensations in your body, such as warmth, heaviness, or lightness. Notice and observe these sensations without judgment or attachment. Additionally, pay attention to your breath, noticing the natural flow of inhalation and exhalation. Let the breath be a source of grounding and relaxation throughout the practice.

7. Visualization and Imagery: Enter a state of profound relaxation by visualizing and experiencing diverse images or scenes in your head. These may include quiet landscapes, serene natural environments, or personal emblems of tranquility. Allow yourself to totally immerse yourself in these visions, using all your senses to experience them vividly.

8. Sankalpa (positive affirmation): At a specific time in the practice, you will be requested to repeat a sankalpa, which is a positive affirmation or vow. Choose a statement that connects with your aim for the practice or any good change you seek in your life. Repeat this sentence silently in your thoughts with conviction, believing in its potential to manifest in your   life.

9. Cultivate Witness Consciousness: Throughout the practice, maintain a sense of witness consciousness. Observe your ideas, feelings, and sensations as they arise without becoming connected to them. Simply

notice their presence and let them pass through, restoring your focus to the practice and the advice.

10. Gradual Awakening: Towards the end of the exercise, you will be guided to gradually awaken your body and bring your awareness back to the present moment. Follow the directions to progressively introduce movement back into your body, wriggling your fingers and toes, stretching softly, and taking a few deep breaths.

11. Reflect and Integrate: After completing the Yoga Nidra exercise, spend a few moments reflecting on your experience. Notice any shifts in your physical body, emotions, or mental condition. Observe the general sense of rest and renewal that you may have cultivated. Allow yourself to thoroughly absorb the advantages of the practice into your being.

12. Practice Regularly: To fully feel the advantages of Yoga Nidra, make it a regular component of your self-care regimen. Aim to practice at least once or twice a week, or as often as feels comfortable for you. Consistency is crucial to increasing your experience and receiving the long-term advantages of this practice

13. Explore Different Guided Recordings or Classes: There are different guided Yoga Nidra recordings and classes available, each with a unique approach and emphasis. Explore numerous possibilities to find a style

that resonates with you. You may find recordings that explicitly target relaxation, stress alleviation, healing, or certain purposes. Experiment and find the ones that deliver you the most joy.

14. Personalize Your Practice: As you grow more experienced with Yoga Nidra, feel free to personalize the practice to meet your needs and tastes. You can combine extra aspects such as quiet music, nature noises, or the use of essential oils to improve the sensory experience. Modify the exercise according to your comfort and make it a truly nourishing and transformational experience for yourself.

15. Seek assistance and support: If you find it beneficial, seek assistance and support from experienced Yoga Nidra practitioners or teachers. They can provide deeper insights, answer your questions, and offer specific assistance to strengthen your practice. Attending workshops or retreats dedicated to Yoga Nidra can also expand your awareness and provide a supportive environment.

Remember that yoga nidra is a practice of deep relaxation and self-discovery. Through regular practice, you can experience profound rejuvenation, reduce stress, enhance sleep quality, and create a greater sense of well-being. Embrace the journey of exploring the ecstasy of Yoga Nidra, and may it bring you to a state of deep relaxation, inner peace, and profound transformation.

Chapter 8

Conclusion

8.1 Embrace the Tranquility Within: The Journey to Lasting Sleep and Relaxation

Congratulations on reaching the end of this inquiry into the power of restful sleep and deep relaxation. Throughout this trip, we have looked into many approaches, practices, and tactics targeted at helping you attain optimal sleep and profound relaxation. By embracing these concepts, you can experience a revolutionary shift in your well-being and overall quality of life.

In this concluding chapter, let us reflect on the important observations and conclusions from our exploration:

1. Sleep and relaxation are vital for overall well-being. Recognize the importance of sleep and relaxation in preserving your physical, mental, and emotional wellness. Prioritize them as vital components of your self-care routine.

2. Mindfulness and meditation are strong tools. Embrace the techniques of mindfulness and meditation to create a peaceful and present frame of

mind. These routines not only increase your sleep but also bring countless benefits to other aspects of your life.

3. Body scan meditation promotes deep relaxation. Utilize the practice of body scan meditation to relieve tension, bring awareness to your body, and induce a state of profound relaxation. This approach allows you to connect with your body and build a harmonious mind-body connection.

4. Guided imagery increases relaxation. Explore the practice of guided imagery, allowing your mind to wander to tranquil and serene places. Through visualization, you can develop a profound sense of relaxation and inner serenity.

5. Progressive muscle relaxation reduces physical stress. Engage in progressive muscle relaxation techniques to methodically release tension from your body. This exercise promotes relaxation, eliminates physical discomfort, and prepares your body for healthy sleep.

6. Sleep hygiene produces a healthy sleep environment: Implement sleep hygiene techniques to maximize your sleep environment. By prioritizing darkness, quietness, a pleasant temperature, and a technology-free zone, you create an atmosphere conducive to restful sleep.

7. Yoga Nidra promotes deep relaxation and rejuvenation. Experience the profound advantages of Yoga Nidra, a practice that combines deep

relaxation and self-awareness. Embrace the step-by-step guide to attain a state of peaceful relaxation and tap into your inner wisdom.

8. Personalize and adapt the practices: Remember that everyone is unique, and it's necessary to personalize and adjust these practices to meet your own needs and preferences. Experiment with different tactics, adapt them as required, and find what resonates with you.

9. Consistency and self-compassion are key. Establishing a consistent schedule and practicing self-compassion are crucial components of this journey. Be patient with yourself, accept the process, and appreciate even the minor accomplishments along the way.

As you end this journey, bring the knowledge, strategies, and practices with you. Integrate them into your daily life, making them a natural part of your self-care regimen. Embrace the peace within you and let it permeate every part of your life.

Remember that the power of restful sleep and deep relaxation lies within your reach. By prioritizing your well-being, nurturing your mind and body, and persistently engaging in these activities, you may uncover the transformational power of tranquility.

8.2 Recap of Key Practices and Techniques

Throughout this book, we have covered a wide range of practices and approaches to foster restful sleep and profound relaxation. As we complete our adventure, let's take a moment to recall some of the significant practices and techniques you have encountered:

1. Mindfulness Meditation: Cultivate present-moment awareness through mindfulness meditation. Practice techniques such as breath awareness, body scan meditation, and mindful breathing to anchor yourself in the present and encourage calm.

2. Guided Imagery: Utilize the power of visualization and guided imagery to create a serene inner environment. Engage your senses and immerse yourself in relaxing landscapes to boost relaxation and invite tranquility.

3. Progressive Muscle Relaxation: Release stress and unwind your body with progressive muscle relaxation. Systematically tense and relax different muscle groups to create profound relaxation and a sensation of ease.

4. Sleep Hygiene: Establish a sleep-friendly environment by prioritizing aspects such as darkness, silence, a pleasant temperature, and minimizing electronic devices. Create a consistent bedtime ritual that

promotes relaxation and communicates to your body that it's time to sleep.

5. Yoga Nidra: Experience deep relaxation and renewal through the practice of Yoga Nidra. Follow guided directions to bring your body and mind into a state of profound serenity while being cognizant and aware.

6. Mindful Breathing: Harness serenity by practicing mindful breathing. Cultivate awareness of your breath by adopting techniques such as deep belly breathing, counting breaths, or alternate nostril breathing to induce relaxation and produce a calm frame of mind.

7. Guided Meditation: Engage in guided meditation recordings or seminars intended exclusively for relaxation and sleep. Follow the instructions and allow yourself to be guided through a journey of inner serenity and tranquility.

8. Sleep Environment Optimization: Create a sleep environment that encourages restful sleep by addressing issues such as light, noise, temperature, and comfort. Make modifications to create darkness, silence, and a calming atmosphere favorable to deep relaxation.

By implementing these practices and techniques into your daily life, you can boost your sleep quality, reduce stress, and foster a state of profound relaxation. Remember that consistency and self-compassion are crucial as you negotiate your particular route toward prolonged sleep and relaxation.

As you move forward, take the time to investigate and personalize these techniques based on your tastes and needs. Listen to your body and honor its messages, allowing yourself the room and grace to adjust and modify your approach as necessary.

Embrace the benefits of peaceful sleep and deep relaxation as a core pillar of your entire well-being. By prioritizing your rest and rejuvenation, you are nurturing your mind, body, and spirit and laying the foundation for a healthy and full life.

May the practices and skills you have learned guide you toward a lifetime of pleasant sleep, great relaxation, and a deep connection with yourself. Embrace the peace within, and may it flow forth, improving every part of your life.

8.3 Embracing a Life of Renewal: Final Thoughts on Sleep and Relaxation

As we come to the close of this trip studying the power of restful sleep and deep relaxation, it is important to reflect on the significant impact these practices may have on our lives. Sleep and relaxation are not only luxury items; they are fundamental components of a healthy and fulfilled existence. By accepting the methods and principles presented in this book, you have taken a huge step towards nourishing your well-being and developing a life of renewal.

Sleep is an essential element of our existence, acting as a time for our bodies to recover, restore, and rejuvenate. It is during sleep that our minds assimilate information, solidify memories, and rejuvenate for the trials and joys of the day ahead. By prioritizing great sleep, we unlock the potential for increased physical health, mental clarity, emotional balance, and overall vitality.

Deep relaxation, on the other hand, allows us to tap into a state of profound tranquility and inner peace, even during our waking hours. Through practices such as mindfulness, meditation, guided imagery, progressive muscle relaxation, and Yoga Nidra, we have explored numerous approaches to achieving this state of peace. These activities give us an opportunity to relieve stress, reduce anxiety, and create a deep sense of connectedness with ourselves and the world around us.

In our modern, fast-paced lives, it is tempting to disregard the value of sleep and relaxation. We typically value productivity and external achievements over our own well-being. However, by choosing a life of renewal, we reclaim our authority to care for ourselves holistically.

Remember that the benefits of sleep and relaxation extend much beyond the time spent in bed or engaged in specific practices. When we prioritize our sleep and make conscious attempts to relax, we generate a ripple effect that favorably benefits every part of our lives.

We become more robust, concentrated, and present. We enjoy better joy, inventiveness, and emotional stability. We build healthier relationships, improved productivity, and a deeper connection with our inner selves.

It is my hope that the knowledge, insights, and practical techniques presented in this book have empowered you to embark on a journey of self-care and regeneration. Embrace the wisdom of restful sleep and deep relaxation as lifetime partners, and let them guide you towards a life filled with vigor, tranquility, and fulfillment.

As you move forward, remember that the journey to optimal sleep and relaxation is ongoing. It demands ongoing self-reflection, modification, and self-compassion. Be open to exploring new techniques, seeking guidance when needed, and refining your routines to correspond with your growing needs and circumstances.

By nourishing your sleep and relaxation, you are investing in your general well-being, happiness, and longevity. Embrace the gift of restoration that sleep and relaxation bring, and allow them to be your allies in living a life of vitality, purpose, and deep fulfillment.

May you find refuge in the embrace of restful sleep and profound relaxation, and may they guide you towards a life of restored energy, balance, and inner harmony.

www.ingramcontent.com/pod-product-compliance
Lightning Source LLC
Chambersburg PA
CBHW051823250726